Coach Kevin's Weight Loss Workbook
by Coach Kevin Trumpfeller

Disclaimer:
This workbook is designed to introduce you to a healthy lifestyle and is intended to help you identify and make healthier choices in nutrition and exercise in order to lose weight safely and effectively.

While I am an experienced Nurse, Certified Health Coach, and Certified Personal Trainer, I am NOT a physician or dietician and this workbook is NOT intended as medical advice or exercise prescription. (Visit the About me tab of my website below to view my qualifications and certifications)

You should discuss your plans to improve your diet and increase your activity level with your Physician before you undertake any new program. This is especially important if you are under a Physician's care for a medical condition or taking prescribed medication! Get that clearance from your Doctor, and let's get started!

If you have questions or concerns, I am available through my website:coachkevintrumpfeller.com or by email at: emailcoachkevin@gmail.com

Coach Kevin Trumpfeller

Hello,

My name is Coach Kevin and welcome to *Coach Kevin's Weight Loss Workbook!* This workbook is designed to guide you through your first 30 days of your weight loss journey.

Together using this workbook we will plan, set goals, and choose healthier foods while we eliminate problem foods and discover why you crave them. Then we'll get you up off that couch and moving more and burning fat and calories - all by following the suggested activities on the following pages...

This workbook is designed as a weight loss activity guide and journal. Once you complete the exercises and activities and then record them - you WILL lose weight.

There are no secrets here, only safe and effective lifestyle changes that result in weight loss. By making a commitment and writing it down, then tracking your progress you will be able to lose weight and keep it off! USE this workbook, and use it every day to make your weight loss dreams a reality.

Before we continue - this workbook is designed as an activity guide and journal, literally a fill in the blanks and worksheets planner and tracking device. For this workbook to be the most effective in helping with your weight loss - you must use it as it is intended. Answer the questions, fill in the blanks, take the time to use the charts and tracking and journal pages!

You are ACCOUNTABLE to this workbook! It is where you will record your weight loss goals and track your progress and success EVERY DAY.

Make a commitment to take the time and make the effort to fill in the blanks and worksheets and to complete the simple tasks required and - you WILL lose weight.

Some of the little things that I ask you to do may seem silly or a waste of time, but there is a reason that I want you to do them... because they have been proven to work.

Some tasks will require painful self-examination and some self-discovery and then writing those things down. No one else needs to see those pages, but YOU DO need to see them and it's important to be honest with yourself in order to move forward and be successful in reaching your weight loss goals.

Are you ready? Let's get started!

Today is ZERO DAY

In order to track your weight loss progress, it's important to know where you began, and that's today - Zero Day.

So, you want to lose weight - and don't we all. Maybe you've tried to lose weight in the past but weren't successful, or maybe you lost the weight but gained it all back.

But this time will be different, this time, you have a Coach (me) and an activity and accountability workbook and journal. I am not there with you to teach, train or motivate you to eat healthier and move more or push you when you get lazy or want to quit...but this Weight Loss Workbook on the table in front of you IS! But you have to USE IT - and use it every day. Commit to it...

Hold your right hand up or place it over your heart and announce to the World, and more importantly, to yourself "I WILL use this Weight Loss Workbook EVERY DAY. I WILL do my best to complete the activities and exercises and record my successes and failures and likes and dislikes and progress EVERY DAY. I WILL keep an open mind and try these new activities, new foods and face these new challenges presented in this workbook and I WILL LOSE WEIGHT!"

Signed _____ Dated _____

ZERO DAY (continued)

Time to take a close look at your weight loss goals. You need to set a specific, realistic and measurable weight loss goal within a specific limited time period. Then you need to WRITE that goal down and work every day to reach it. That's what this Weight Loss Workbook is designed to help you do.

Maybe you need to lose 30, 50 or 100 pounds...it is doable, but let's save those for intermediate and long-term goals. This workbook is designed for 30 days, so let's set a short-term goal for the next 30 day period. A good (safe and sustainable) weight loss goal for 30 days would be 10-15 pounds. So, how about 10 pounds in the next 30 days? Too little? Not really, 10 pounds in safe and sustainable and permanent weight loss would result in a total 30 pounds lost in 3 months, sound better? Would losing 30 pounds improve your life?

YOUR FIRST GOAL: I WILL LOSE _____lbs./kgs

in the next 30 DAYS! I WILL LOSE THIS WEIGHT BECAUSE:

Signed _____ Dated _____

Good job! Your goal is clear, realistic and measurable.

ZERO DAY (continued)

Look back at your first goal, what was the reason that you put just below it? Why do you want to lose weight? Find a reason, or a bunch of reasons why you WANT to lose the weight. Not reasons that you HAVE TO. You are much more likely to reach goals that involve things (reasons) that you WANT. For example, I WANT to buy new clothes, I WANT to fit into and wear my wedding dress, I want everyone to be jealous of my new slim and trim figure in that new swimsuit on the beach in Hawaii...get the idea?

I WANT to lose weight because:

Good job! Now you understand your motivation.

ZERO DAY (continued)

The final thing we need to do on ZERO DAY is to record your weight and take measurements to track your progress and to compare with your final weight and measurements at the end of your first 30 days. NO one need see these measurements, but it is easier if a second person handles the tape measure for you.

Today is _____

I am _____ Tall and Weigh _____

My Neck at the widest point is _____

My Chest measures _____

My Waist at the widest point is _____

My Hips measure _____

My Left Thigh _____ My Left Calf _____

My Left Upper Arm _____ My Left Forearm _____

Optional: My calculated BMI is _____

Optional: Photos were taken _____Yes _____No

My Weight Loss Goal Sheet

I, _____

WILL LOSE _____pounds/kilograms

BEFORE _____ 20_____

I WILL SUCCESSFULLY LOSE THIS WEIGHT BECAUSE:

_____

_____

_____

_____

_____

_____

SIGNED _____ DATE _____

Witness (optional)_____

Post one copy on your refrigerator, mirror and one in your purse or pocket!

My Weight Loss Goal Sheet

I, _____

WILL LOSE _____pounds/kilograms

BEFORE _____ 20_____

I WILL SUCCESSFULLY LOSE THIS WEIGHT BECAUSE:

_____

_____

_____

_____

_____

_____

SIGNED _____ DATE _____

Witness (optional)_____

Post one copy on your refrigerator, mirror and one in your purse or pocket!

My Weight Loss Goal Sheet

I, _____

WILL LOSE _____pounds/kilograms

BEFORE _____ 20_____

I WILL SUCCESSFULLY LOSE THIS WEIGHT BECAUSE:

_____

_____

_____

_____

_____

SIGNED _____ DATE _____

Witness (optional)_____

Post one copy on your refrigerator, mirror and one in your purse or pocket!

We all know that dieting is difficult.

Your pants are too tight, your zipper won't close, and the scale seems to be out of control. And dieting for women seems even more difficult, but healthy lifestyle changes including proper diet and exercise are not only possible but critical for safe and lasting weight loss.

You've tried those yo-yo fad diets and now it's time to get serious and make some healthy lifestyle changes including cleaning up your diet and moving more.

When you hear the word "diet" what comes to mind? Probably an unpleasant and unhappy calorie restricted attempt to lose weight. But your "diet" is actually the total of the foods that you eat, although we often use the term to describe our weight loss "plans" good or bad.

But, which diet is best for you? The best diet for you will always be the one that you'll follow and stick to. But whatever diet you follow, remember that it's important to get all of the nutrients your body needs, and unfortunately, diets that restrict a particular food category make this difficult.

Before we discuss diets and eating plans, it's very important to understand body fat and fat storage. Once you understand why your body stores fat, you can take the necessary steps to defeat the fat storage cycle.

Humans store fat in their bodies as a primitive means of survival. Our ancestors lived from one meal to the next, they were hunters and gatherers who did not always know where their next meal was coming from. During the "feast" times, their bodies would convert calories into stored energy as fat in order to better survive the "famine" periods until that next meal became available.

Unfortunately for us, we now live in constant feast periods with an overly abundant supply of food and our bodies continue to store (and stockpile) fat supplies for the famine period that may never come.

And to make matters worse, if we consciously decide to shed some of that stored fat by dieting, our bodies interpret that restriction of food and calories as "famine" and will do everything it can to hold on to that emergency fat supply.

When you diet, your body will literally fight you to keep from losing the stored energy (fat) that it thinks is necessary for your future survival.

What can we learn from this?

Don't skip meals. If you skip a meal or meals, your body releases hormones to promote fat storage. Your body goes into a temporary starvation mode, slows your metabolism and holds on to the fat for survival. How can you lose fat by restricting calories if every time that you do you body works harder to keep that fat?

You can't. Restricting calories and skipping meals will always cause that survival fat storage cycle to kick in. The best way to combat that cycle is by eating smaller, healthier and more frequent meals, drinking more water, and moving more to increase your fat-burning metabolism.

OK, the lecture is over for today, let's do some real work.

Today is DAY 1. Before we make any radical changes, let's look at your current diet and lifestyle. A simple exercise to help you see what you eat and drink all day, every day.

Use the following page (or pages if you need them) to record the foods you eat, the times you eat and the beverages you drink.

Be honest, no one will see this unless you show them and the list will be useful very soon. DO NOT worry about calories, but times, frequency and general serving sizes are important.

Try to record your drinks as well, if you drink colas, sodas, etc. record the sizes like 16oz. or 1 Liter, etc.

Be as accurate as you can be, and don't change your diet for this day just because you know that you will be recording it here. We are looking for foods and patterns that we can improve on in the next few days to help you make healthier choices to help you lose that weight!

Healthy Activity #1 Date:_____

Time: _____ Foods:_____
_____
_____
_____
Drinks: _____
_____
_____

Time: _____ Foods:_____
_____
_____
Drinks: _____
_____
_____

Time: _____ Foods:_____
_____
_____
Drinks: _____
_____
_____

Any thoughts about what's on this list? _____
_____
_____
_____

Healthy Activity #1 Food Diary (continued)

Time: _____ Foods: _____
_____
_____

Drinks: _____
_____
_____

Time: _____ Foods: _____
_____
_____

Drinks: _____
_____
_____

Time: _____ Foods: _____
_____
_____

Drinks: _____
_____
_____

Any thoughts about what's on this list? _____
_____
_____
_____

Did you notice anything about the foods that you eat as you wrote them down or now that you see them listed?

_____ How many are fast foods or prepackaged convenience foods?

_____ How many carbonated colas or sodas?

_____ How many bottled juices or syrupy coffees?

_____ How much time between your meals or snacks?

_____ How many snacks and what type?

_____ How much water did you drink? Milk?

_____ How many burgers, fries, slices of pizza?

_____ Did you notice how much salad dressing or condiments like ketchup (catsup) you used?

_____ How many slices of bread, tortillas, or bagels?

_____ How many sweets, desserts, added sugar?

Do you notice any patterns? Any changes that you could make on your own? _____

Make Healthier Choices: Drink More Water

The first step to safe and permanent weight loss is to make healthier choices. You will soon be choosing more fresh and wholesome foods to replace the processed fast foods and prepackaged convenience foods that we all turn to when we are in a hurry or stressed.

We'll talk more about food choices tomorrow, but today, I want you to focus on drinking more water. It doesn't have to be fancy or expensive bottled water (although some of the commercially available filtered and purified waters are healthier than tap water).

Replacing all the liquid sugar, syrupy coffee concoctions, bottled juices and carbonated colas with water is one of the easiest and most effective steps you can take to better health. Drink plenty of WATER, fresh clean water.

Drink another glass of water 30 minutes before each meal and you will eat less and consume fewer calories. The more water you drink, the fewer calories you'll consume and feel full longer. Drinking more water will also help your body flush and eliminate the fat from your system.

Instead of drinking soda, alcoholic beverages, juices, or other high-calorie drinks, grab a glass or bottle of water. Choosing a zero-calorie beverage over high-calorie drinks can spare you hundreds of calories per day, boosting your weight loss!

Healthy Activity #2   Water Tips and Calculations

Let's calculate how much water you should drink every day: If you measure your weight in pounds, divide your weight by 2 and drink that many ounces of water daily.

For example, if you weigh 160 pounds / 2 = 80 ounces. In this example, you would drink 80 ounces over the course of the day. Sounds like a lot, but it is really only 10 small 8 ounce cups or juice glasses. Easy.

Now do your calculations:

Divide your estimated ounces over the entire day. Have your first glass as soon as you wake up and another with lemon juice at breakfast. Fresh lemon juice in your water will add flavor and also improves kidney and liver function.

Track your water intake today:

_____ Glass 1 _____ Glass 2 _____Glass 3

_____ Glass 4 _____ Glass 5 _____Glass 6

_____ Glass 7 _____ Glass 8 _____Glass 9

We're all busy with LIFE and we don't often think about the health benefits (or unhealthy consequences) of the foods we eat. Sadly, eating healthy isn't a priority or part of our normal daily routine. But healthy eating is something we should be concerned about every day. Our modern diet consists primarily of high fat, high sugar, and high sodium foods that are mostly pre-packaged, overly processed, and of the fast-food (junk) variety.

A body fueled by junk food, fast food, convenience food and processed foods and sugar soon becomes fat, sick, and tired. Check your local library or search the internet for Morgan Spurlock's 2004 classic documentary and social experiment in fast-food: Super Size Me. Although produced over 10 years ago, it is still relevant today and it will change how you look at junk food and fast food.

Eating healthy, natural whole food can give you more energy, improve performance and mental alertness and build stronger bones, and leaner muscles!

Take the first step and add fruits and vegetables to your diet. Choose lean proteins from free-range and grass-fed meats and wild fish, add beans and whole unprocessed grains. Today is a good day to begin eliminating those toxic hormone and antibiotic-laden dairy products, over-refined and processed grains and sugars. Take the first step toward eating healthy and you'll soon see a happier and healthier YOU!

Healthy Activity #3 Adding Fruit to Your Diet

Make a list of fruits you enjoy: _____

_____

_____

_____

_____

How many of those are in your kitchen right now? _____

_____

Why is that? _____

What are we going to do about it? _____

Your answer should be - go to the store or market and buy fruit. If your favorite fresh fruits aren't available, buy frozen or packaged fruit (packed in juice, NOT syrup). Find ways to add fruit to your diet, then find ways to use fruit as a healthy snack, finally, look for ways to replace unhealthy foods or sweets with fruit.

Soon we will be replacing entire meals with easy to prepare healthy smoothies made by tossing available fruits and vegetables into your blender.   - Eat more FRUIT!

HELLO! HAVE YOU NOTICED

THAT THE BACK OF YOUR

WEIGHT LOSS WORKBOOK

IS FILLED WITH ALL KINDS OF

DAILY JOURNAL AND DIARY PAGES?

USE THEM EVERY DAY TO TRACK

YOUR WEIGHT LOSS PROGRESS

AND ACTIVITY FOR 30 DAYS.

START TODAY!

Healthy Activity #4 Your Kitchen Photo Overview

Before we make any serious changes to your diet and the foods that you currently eat, let's "take stock" and make a photographic record so that you can reflect back on "the old days and old ways" before you lost weight and started eating healthy.

Whip out your cell phone or digital camera and open your cabinet doors, your refrigerator and freezer and start on one side of the kitchen and click away until you photograph the entire open display. Now you have a digital history of how you used to eat. Record the date: _____

What do you notice about the foods in your cabinets or pantry? _____
_____

Are there many boxes of cookies, cereals, sugar, white flour, bread, toaster pastries, bags of chips? _____

How about that refrigerator? What do you see right up front? What do you reach for first? Healthy foods? _____
_____

And the freezer? Frozen pizzas, frozen dinners and ice cream containers? _____

What are we going to do about it? _____
_____

If you really want to lose weight and improve your lifestyle by making healthier choices, you'll start by throwing those foods that you know are garbage - in the garbage.

OR, bag them up and donate them to a friend, relative, some type of charity or mission or shelter...

OR, at the very least, if you can't afford that option or just can't bear the thought of wasting food (like me) promise that as you use up and empty each unhealthy food you will replace it with a leaner, healthier option!

"I PROMISE THAT WHEN THE COOKIES ARE GONE, NO MORE!_____(initials)

"I PROMISE THAT WHEN THE CHIPS, SODAS, ICE CREAM, PIZZAS, WHITE BREAD AND PASTRIES ARE GONE, I WON'T BUY MORE!" _____(initials)

"YES, I AM SERIOUS ABOUT LOSING WEIGHT. YES, I WANT TO LOSE POUNDS AND INCHES AND I WANT TO DO IT NOW!" and "THAT'S WHY THIS JUNK FOOD & GARBAGE HAS TO GO!" Sign it:_____
Date it: _____   Now DO IT!

To make the kinds of changes that you WANT to make in your life, in your appearance, in your health and happiness, you will have to make sacrifices and give up some of the foods and drinks that got you where you are. Period.

Throw out the garbage - and don't look back.

"OK," you say, "I really do want to lose weight and improve my health and happiness, but how do I know what's garbage, and what's food and what to eat...it's all so confusing. Can you help me understand?"

Yes, it can be confusing, so many people tell you so many different things and that you should eat this and don't eat that and then the people who manufacture your "food" tell you something entirely different. "Be Happy - Enjoy _____ "

Not to be completely cynical or some kind of conspiracy theorist, but those 'nice' folks who make your food, put it in the can or bottle your bubbly drinks or flip your burgers or slide your pizza into the box, those people DO NOT CARE about you or your health or your waistline.

They only care about SALES and PROFIT. And if it TASTES GOOD, if it's sweet or salty, or hot and greasy - that sells more "food". Unfortunately, sweet requires TOO MUCH sugar just as salty requires TOO MUCH salt, see the pattern? A little is OK, but we want MORE, so the people who make our food give us MORE! And we buy it, eat it, and get fat and sick. Obesity, diabetes, hypertension, heart disease and even some forms of cancer are caused by or complicated by the pre-packaged, overly processed and convenience fast foods that we eat every day.

OK, rant over. But for the next thirty days during your weight loss journey, THINK about everything you eat and drink - as you eat it....is it really good for you? WHY are you eating it? Is it the healthiest choice you could make?

Making healthy food choices does require a very BASIC understanding of nutrition the foods we eat and can help you make healthier choices in the grocery store and the kitchen. You're probably already familiar with the terms fat, protein, and carbohydrates (carbs) which are examples of "macronutrients". Macronutrients provide calories and energy and micronutrients are the vitamins and minerals.

Carbohydrates
There are three types of carbohydrates (or carbs) - sugar, starch, and fiber. Sugars are simple carbohydrates while starches and dietary fiber are considered complex carbohydrates. Simple carbohydrates are also known as fast (or fast-acting) carbs as they cause an almost immediate rise in blood sugar. Complex carbohydrates or slow carbs are more difficult to digest and absorb and do not cause rapid spikes in blood sugar levels.

Proteins
Our bodies use protein to build and repair muscle tissues and to produce enzymes and hormones. Protein provides the necessary building blocks for bones, tendons and cartilage, skin and nails, and is crucial for the production of hemoglobin in our blood.

Proteins contain complex compounds called amino acids. Essential amino acids come only from the foods that we eat, and only animal sources of protein provide all of the essential amino acids that we need. Animal proteins are said to be nutritionally complete.

Fats

Fats are said to be either saturated or unsaturated. Saturated fats are fat molecules saturated with hydrogen molecules. You can recognize saturated fats as they are usually solid at room temperature.

Examples would include animal fat, butter, cheese and ice cream.

Unsaturated Fats are usually liquid at room temperature and are primarily from fish, vegetable sources and oils. Unsaturated fats also contain fatty acids (omega-3 fatty acids) which are considered "healthy" fats as they promote heart health and lower cholesterol.

Sources include fish oil, avocado, olive oil and oils from nuts and seeds.

Trans Fats are a type of fat that are man-made and produced from chemicals in a laboratory. Trans fats are dangerous and have been shown to cause diseases including heart disease and cancer.

Most food manufacturers are voluntarily removing trans fats from their products and are required to clearly label foods containing trans fats.

Trans fats should be avoided at all cost.

Healthy Activity #5 Making Healthy Choices

Making healthy food choices does not have to be complicated. Start by adding fresh fruits and vegetables along with lean protein from free-range and grass-fed meats and wild fish, beans, and whole grains. Choose organic products when available and begin eliminating toxic hormones and antibiotic-enhanced dairy products, over-refined and processed grains and sugars.

Learn to read food labels and make the healthiest choices and you'll be rewarded with more energy, improved performance and a stronger, leaner body.

What Proteins do you eat? _____

_____

_____

_____

How about Carbohydrates? _____

_____

_____

_____

_____

And Fats?_____

_____

_____

_____

Making Healthy Choices (continued)

This activity involves HOMEWORK, RESEARCH and a FIELD TRIP to your local grocery store. Search books, magazines and the internet for HEALTHY FOODS. List them here and search for them where you shop for groceries. We'll compare lists in the workbook sections that follow.

What Proteins SHOULD you eat? _____

_____

_____

_____

_____

_____

What Carbohydrates SHOULD you eat? _____

_____

_____

_____

_____

_____

_____

What healthy Fats SHOULD you eat? (hint: Avocados should be on this list) _____

_____

_____

_____

_____

_____

Here is MY list, but keep in mind that it is VERY RESTRICTIVE and may be too extreme for your first month of Healthy Eating. But look for these items in your local store and find products similar to those listed below. Think of it as a Healthy Scavenger Hunt.

Coach Kevin's Sample Healthy GROCERY LIST

Breads: Ezekiel brand bread (in the freezer section). Alvarado Street Bakery brand bread and rolls.
If you have a Trader Joe's, look for the store brand whole grain bread, and try their Sprouted Multi-Grain bread and California Protein bread.

Crackers: Look for Ak-Mak Whole Wheat Crackers.

Tortillas: Look for tortillas made from organic (GMO-free) corn, lime, and water or a sprouted wheat tortilla.

Dairy & Non-Dairy: Try an organic, full-fat milk. Use organic full-fat milk as a fat and carbohydrate, not a protein. The lower the fat content of your milk, the more processed that milk is. Used in moderation, full fat milk is healthier than 2%.

Cottage cheese: Full fat is best, but you can also use low fat. (but NOT fat-free)

Yogurt: Always choose plain Greek yogurt. And mix in your own fresh fruits and a few drops of honey or a natural sweetener if you need it flavored. Choose full-fat over reduced or non-fat.

Cheese: Buy REAL cheese. Don't buy shredded cheese as it's coated with unhealthy anti-caking agents. Buy block cheese and slice or shred it yourself.

Try unsweetened almond milk you may prefer it over dairy. You may want to try unsweetened rice milk or unsweetened soy milk, or unsweetened coconut milk.

Eggs: Choose free range and cage free eggs if they are available.

Chicken & Turkey: Boneless, skinless poultry breasts are good choices. If you can find and afford organic, it's always a better choice.

Beef: Choose grass fed and free range beef. If you need help, your butcher can help you choose the best cuts. If you are open to new things, try venison and bison.

Pork: Choose lean cuts of pork. Ask your butcher for help. Avoid fatty and processed pork products like ham, bacon and sausage.

Fish can be a healthy choice, but choose farm-raised fish or fish that is most likely free from mercury and heavy metals.

Oatmeal: Choose plain oatmeal, not the flavored varieties. Steel cut oats or traditional rolled oats are best.

Dried beans and legumes: Lentils, black beans or chickpeas.

Load up on Fruits and Vegetables (fresh if available):
Apples
Oranges
Grapefruits
Banana
Avocados
Berries of all kinds
Cherries
Kiwi
And any other fresh or frozen fruit that you enjoy.

Vegetables:
Carrots
Celery
Spinach
Broccoli
Bell Peppers (any color)
Zucchini
Eggplant
Squash of any variety
Kale
Chard
Collard greens
Okra
Green beans
Tomatoes
Sweet potatoes
Onions (any variety)
And any other fresh or frozen vegetables that you will eat.

HAVE YOU COMPLETED YOUR DAILY JOURNAL AND DIARY PAGES?

USE THEM EVERY DAY TO TRACK YOUR WEIGHT LOSS PROGRESS DIET AND ACTIVITY FOR 30 DAYS.

DO IT NOW!

Let's talk about exercise...

Exercise and healthy eating are the two most important steps that you can take to LOSE WEIGHT and improve your health. Exercise can also improve your circulation, relieve stress and decrease your risk of heart disease.

But if you're new to exercise or haven't exercised in years, it's important to ease into it in order to prevent muscle soreness or injury. Yes, you really do have to walk before you can run. Remember, before you start your new exercise program, you should talk to your family physician and explain that you are planning to increase your activity level. Once you're cleared, it's time to get started.

You should always warm up your muscles and gently stretch before beginning your exercise sessions, and don't forget to drink plenty of water no matter what exercise program you choose to follow whether at home, at the nearest public school track or your local gym.

But, if the thought of exercise scares you or you're not quite ready to join that big gym or exercise in public in your bright new shiny shoes and neon shorts, there is an alternative...

But first, you must commit to increasing your activity level and get off your butt and off that couch and start moving! Come on, it only takes 30 minutes of activity to get that metabolism buzzing!

Stop using that "I don't have time to exercise" excuse. If you have time to stream Netflix movies, or socialize on Facebook, or play video games, you have plenty of time to exercise.

Here are some ideas to get you off the couch and increase your activity level without actually "exercising":

Get OUTSIDE and start walking! Walk to the grocery store, walk until the dog is tired, walk to the drugstore, Post Office, local school, or the Library. Work up to walking 30 minutes every day at a brisk pace and if you can't, then walk in 10-minute time chunks.

Clean your house. Clean at least one room every day thoroughly and VIGOROUSLY. After you've cleaned them all, do it again. You can easily burn 300-400 calories vacuuming and straightening just one room daily. Once you are done or the task becomes too easy, add additional tasks like laundry and ironing.

Set a timer for 30 minutes and work until it goes off. That's 30 minutes of continuous activity (exercise) without even thinking about it.

Do you have a treadmill out in the garage or gathering dust somewhere? Drag that treadmill in front of your television and I mean directly in front of the screen so that you have to be WALKING on it to watch that reality show or whatever it is that you really want to watch. Up, OFF the couch and MOVING in the privacy of your own home.

Do you like to dance? Lock the front door, crank up your favorite music and dance till you can't dance anymore. Thirty minutes minimum and feel much better for it.

Find some kids, either your own or borrow them if you have to, and throw a ball, throw a frisbee or chase each other around in the park. Play tag, push the swing, hide-and-seek.

Wash and WAX the car! Push the lawn mower, trim the bushes, clean the pool. Paint the house, redecorate. DIY your entire house. Keep moving, drink water and then do more.

Are you addicted to video games? Use that expensive game system for "exercise" with Wii Fit or Xbox Fitness. There are many new options that require agility and movement. More like playing games than exercising and once you become proficient, challenge your friends and family and get them involved as well!

Make moving fun and challenging and you will look forward to your "exercise" sessions every day. Once these activities become a part of your daily routine, you will find that they become easier each time you do them.

Eventually, you will find yourself looking for new fitness challenges and you will be ready to try the gym or those laps at the local track. But, until then, get off your butt and MOVE for 30 minutes every day!

Time for an Exercise - Exercise...

Healthy Exercise #6 - Your Exercise Choices

From the previous suggestions, let's make a list of exercise ideas that would get your butt off the couch and moving:

Now, pick one. _____
Find some type of timer, set it for 30 minutes and GO!

What are 3 exercise options NOT on the list that you would like to try in the future? What activities would you enjoy?

Once you become more fit, you may want to try more traditional exercise programs, but what exercises should you do? A balanced fitness program should include three types of training: Cardio (Aerobics), Strength, and Flexibility.

Cardiovascular exercise, often shortened to "cardio" promotes good health by training and strengthening the cardio-respiratory system, especially the heart and lungs. Cardio training is considered "aerobic" meaning with oxygen as correct cardio training involves working large muscle groups for an adequate amount of time to increase your heart rate and breathing - both result in increased oxygen consumption (respiratory rate) and distribution (heart rate).

Cardio training requires moving large muscle groups over an extended period of time and requires your body to burn calories. Examples include walking (long or brisk) dancing, jogging, running or bicycle riding.

Strength Training: Using your body weight or weight training (using dumbbells or barbells) is necessary to improve muscle tone and strength. Strength training can also promote the "training effect" and promote additional weight loss and fat burning.

Start with light weights and add weight and reps as you improve. If following a bodyweight program, start with fewer reps and increase as you become stronger.

Flexibility Training: As we grow older our flexibility decreases and our susceptibility to strains, pulled muscles and injuries increases. Flexibility training is often overlooked and underutilized. But, stretching before and after your cardio and strength training sessions will reduce your risk for injury.

Use gentle stretches and no bouncing, slow steady motions combined with gentle breathing... breath and hold. Release and repeat. Flexibility training reduces injury, decreases muscle soreness, and increases the range of motion of your joints, increases muscle coordination, and circulation.

Which types of exercise appeal to you? _____

_____

_____

Do you need to consider joining a gym or studio? _____

What is stopping you? _____

_____

_____

What can you do to overcome these obstacles? _____

_____

Our time together is drawing to a close, but there are a few more subjects that I would like to discuss that have been beneficial in my healthy lifestyle. The first is SMOOTHIES as a meal replacement.

You can take almost any healthy but disgusting vegetable, toss it in your blender and cover it with your favorite fruit and a banana, add some water or any type of milk or milk substitute, add a few ice cubes and blend until smooth and you end up with a Healthy and Nutritious and DELICIOUS shake for breakfast, or post workout refresher or between meal snack!

Do you need some fancy $300 blender? No, use the one you got for a wedding present or the one down under the sink. If the blender you own will crush ice, it will make smoothies. Once you try a few and gain experience and confidence, you will be blending up your own nutritious smoothies. Try them.

Now, I'd like to talk about a simple but highly effective approach to PORTION CONTROL. We've discussed the need to eat smaller and more frequent meals in order to avoid triggering that fat storing "survival" mode.

While you're eating those smaller meals more frequently, eat them in smaller healthier portions. Simple portion control can reduce the total number of calories you consume at every meal and over the course of the day. Use a smaller plate and smaller bowl to trick your brain into thinking those portions are not smaller.

Avoid stress. When you are stressed, you are much more prone to stress eating and stress eating involves lots of sugar and empty calories. The stress of normal daily living naturally decreases hormones and neurotransmitters in our brains.

Unfortunately, your body tries to correct this deficiency by craving sugar. When you eat sugar, your brain releases dopamine and endorphins, the neurotransmitters that cause you to feel "happy".

When we are stressed or unhappy, we turn to foods that make us happy - sugar. Learn to avoid and manage stress in order to avoid the resulting stress eating.

These are the things that stress me OUT! _____
_____
_____
_____
_____
_____
_____

These are things that I can do to relieve that stress! _____
_____
_____
_____
_____
_____
_____
_____without stress eating!

Develop a Support System.

Find friends, relatives, and coworkers who understand and support your need to make these healthy lifestyle changes. Use your new weight loss support group to share tips and experiences, successes and to discuss and overcome challenges.

My Weight Loss Support System includes: _____

_____

_____

_____

_____

_____

_____

_____

_____

Coach Kevin Trumpfeller - coachkevintrumpfeller.com
or contact me by email - emailcoachkevin@gmail.com

CONGRATULATIONS for making it this far! We all have good intentions...but we rarely follow through. We start with good intentions, but then life gets in the way, doesn't it?

Wouldn't it be great to make those healthy nutrition and fitness goals more than dreams and wishes? To LOSE the weight that you dream of losing?

Our daily lives are already a series of habits that we often blindly follow throughout the day…every day. But habits can be changed, as difficult as that seems. Bad habits can be eliminated and good ones can take their place.

If you want to make a better life by including new and healthy habits, the best thing to do is to make small, incremental changes every day. It generally takes about 30 days to change a habit, if you're focused and consistent.

Tell EVERYONE about your new habit. Hey, starting TODAY, I now exercise 30 minutes every morning! Ask for their support. It also helps keep you on track because tomorrow you have to look them in the eye and confirm, YES, I DID do my 30 minutes!

Start NOW! Start today, if possible, tomorrow morning at the latest. No more procrastination...tell yourself it's only a 30-day trial. Start now, and build momentum.

Commit to and stick with your new healthy habits for 30 days, and they become Healthy Habits for LIFE!

How To Maintain Your Weight Loss

Congratulations! You've lost the weight and reached your goal...but don't celebrate too soon. Unfortunately 95% of successful dieters gain that weight back within one year.

Let's take a look at some steps that you can take to keep the weight off. You worked your butt off to take that weight off, isn't it worth the effort to keep it off? Here are a few quick tips:

Don't avoid the scale. If your daily weigh-in was a part of your successful weight loss, don't stop monitoring and tracking your weight now that you have reached your goal. That's not to say you have to step on the scale EVERY day if you did not do that before the weight loss. Weigh in AT LEAST once per week. But, if you weigh 2 or 3 pounds more today than you did three days ago, you did something wrong over that three days. Identify the "rebound" behavior and correct it.

Don't get lazy. What activities and exercises did you do to get to your goal weight? Don't stop now. If you stop or cut back your activity level, your metabolism will slow down. If you continue at least 30 minutes of moderate exercise 3-5 times each week, you will maintain your weight loss and may continue to slim down. If you dread your previous workout program, change it up, try new things, join a gym, train for a race or buy a new bicycle. Set new fitness goals and keep that heart pumping.

Check your emotions. Mood swings, sadness, and depression lead to emotional eating. Similar to the stress eating cause and effect, eating sugar or comfort foods makes us happy or takes us back to happier times during our childhood. Are there certain foods you turn to when you are angry, sad or depressed? Be careful, one episode of emotional eating can lead to serious binge eating and quickly destroy your hard fought gains.

Avoid treats. We are not puppies, why do we reward success and good behavior with "treats"? It starts when we are toddlers and progresses as we age, candy, cookies, cake and ice cream. Stop rewarding yourself (and celebrating) with junk.

Celebrate your successes with a good meal, a new purse, shoes or jewelry. It's not too late to save your own children from this self-destructive practice although you might have to convince YOUR parents that it's the right thing to do.

Take the time. We are all busy in our daily lives. Too busy to shop, cook and prepare healthy meals. We grab something "on the way" to wherever we are going. Fast food, junk food and pre-packaged calorie bombs.

Take the time to shop for and prepare healthy meals (and snacks). Avoid the drive-up windows and talking clowns, they will ruin your weight loss successes!

This section completes the lecture portion of your Weight Loss Workshop. By now, you should have completed all of the Healthy Activities worksheets.

You should have:

_____ Identified and written your weight loss goals.
_____ Explained the reasons WHY you want to lose weight.
_____ POSTED copies of your written goals.
_____ Recorded your weight and beginning measurements.
_____ Listed the foods and drinks that you normally eat.
_____ Evaluated that list of foods and drinks.
_____ Identified healthier foods that you SHOULD eat.
_____ Listed which fruits to add to your diet.
_____ Taken photos of your "before" cabinets and fridge.
_____ Evaluated the GARBAGE foods in your kitchen.
_____ Swore an Oath to get rid of that garbage.
_____ Calculated the amount of water you SHOULD drink.
_____ Made a practice run to the store with your new list.
_____ Identified ways to move more and exercise.
_____ Identified how to handle stress without eating.
_____ Identified your Weight Loss support system.
_____ You've even considered joining a GYM!

Wow, you've been busy!
Now it's time to put your new Healthy Eating, Shopping, and Cooking skills to work. It's also time to Exercise and MOVE more, try a few smoothies and complete the 30-day supply of Weight Loss Worksheets and Journals that follow. GOOD LUCK and GOOD HEALTH!

Coach Kevin

Weight Loss Worksheet for _____ 20_____

Today is Day _____ of 30 and I weigh _____ at _____ am/pm

I have completed a total of _____ minutes of exercise
Including _____
_____

I have eliminated the following garbage food from my diet:
_____
_____

I have replaced the junk with these healthier food choices:
_____
_____

I am particularly proud of Today's accomplishments:
_____
_____

And the ways that I handled stress: _____
_____
_____

But I am REALLY craving: _____
_____

Probably because: _____
_____
_____

My Food Journal for _____ 20_____

Breakfast: _____ AM/PM home/work/school/car/other
I had _____
_____
Proud that I DID NOT have: _____

Snack #1: _____ AM/PM home/work/school/car/other
I had _____
_____
Proud that I DID NOT have: _____

Lunch: _____ AM/PM home/work/school/car/other
I had _____
_____
Proud that I DID NOT have: _____

Snack #2: _____ AM/PM home/work/school/car/other
I had _____
_____
Proud that I DID NOT have: _____

Dinner: _____ AM/PM home/work/school/car/other
I had _____
_____
Proud that I DID NOT have: _____

Drank ___1 ___2 ___3 ___4 ___5 ___6 ___7 ___8 glasses of water!

And feel GOOD about: _____
_____

Weight Loss Worksheet for _____ 20_____

Today is Day _____ of 30 and I weigh _____ at _____ am/pm

I have completed a total of _____ minutes of exercise
Including _____
_____

I have eliminated the following garbage food from my diet:
_____
_____

I have replaced the junk with these healthier food choices:
_____
_____

I am particularly proud of Today's accomplishments:
_____
_____

And the ways that I handled stress: _____
_____
_____

But I am REALLY craving: _____
_____

Probably because: _____
_____
_____

My Food Journal for _____ 20_____

Breakfast: _____ AM/PM home/work/school/car/other
I had _____
_____
Proud that I DID NOT have: _____

Snack #1: _____ AM/PM home/work/school/car/other
I had _____
_____
Proud that I DID NOT have: _____

Lunch: _____ AM/PM home/work/school/car/other
I had _____
_____
Proud that I DID NOT have: _____

Snack #2: _____ AM/PM home/work/school/car/other
I had _____
_____
Proud that I DID NOT have: _____

Dinner: _____ AM/PM home/work/school/car/other
I had _____
_____
Proud that I DID NOT have: _____

Drank ___1 ___2 ___3 ___4 ___5 ___6 ___7 ___8 glasses of water!

And feel GOOD about: _____
_____

Weight Loss Worksheet for _____ 20_____

Today is Day _____ of 30 and I weigh _____ at _____ am/pm

I have completed a total of _____ minutes of exercise
Including _____
_____

I have eliminated the following garbage food from my diet:
_____
_____

I have replaced the junk with these healthier food choices:
_____
_____

I am particularly proud of Today's accomplishments:
_____
_____

And the ways that I handled stress: _____
_____
_____

But I am REALLY craving: _____
_____

Probably because: _____
_____
_____

My Food Journal for _____ 20_____

Breakfast: _____ AM/PM home/work/school/car/other
I had _____
_____
Proud that I DID NOT have: _____

Snack #1: _____ AM/PM home/work/school/car/other
I had _____
_____
Proud that I DID NOT have: _____

Lunch: _____ AM/PM home/work/school/car/other
I had _____
_____
Proud that I DID NOT have: _____

Snack #2: _____ AM/PM home/work/school/car/other
I had _____
_____
Proud that I DID NOT have: _____

Dinner: _____ AM/PM home/work/school/car/other
I had _____
_____
Proud that I DID NOT have: _____

Drank ___1 ___2 ___3 ___4 ___5 ___6 ___7 ___8 glasses of water!

And feel GOOD about: _____
_____

Weight Loss Worksheet for _____ 20_____

Today is Day _____ of 30 and I weigh _____ at _____ am/pm

I have completed a total of _____ minutes of exercise
Including _____
_____

I have eliminated the following garbage food from my diet:
_____
_____

I have replaced the junk with these healthier food choices:
_____
_____

I am particularly proud of Today's accomplishments:
_____
_____

And the ways that I handled stress: _____
_____
_____

But I am REALLY craving: _____
_____

Probably because: _____
_____
_____

My Food Journal for _____ 20_____

Breakfast: _____ AM/PM home/work/school/car/other
I had _____
_____
Proud that I DID NOT have: _____

Snack #1: _____ AM/PM home/work/school/car/other
I had _____
_____
Proud that I DID NOT have: _____

Lunch: _____ AM/PM home/work/school/car/other
I had _____
_____
Proud that I DID NOT have: _____

Snack #2: _____ AM/PM home/work/school/car/other
I had _____
_____
Proud that I DID NOT have: _____

Dinner: _____ AM/PM home/work/school/car/other
I had _____
_____
Proud that I DID NOT have: _____

Drank ___1 ___2 ___3 ___4 ___5 ___6 ___7 ___8 glasses of water!

And feel GOOD about: _____
_____

Weight Loss Worksheet for _____ 20_____

Today is Day _____ of 30 and I weigh _____ at _____ am/pm

I have completed a total of _____ minutes of exercise
Including _____
_____

I have eliminated the following garbage food from my diet:
_____
_____

I have replaced the junk with these healthier food choices:
_____
_____

I am particularly proud of Today's accomplishments:
_____
_____

And the ways that I handled stress: _____
_____
_____

But I am REALLY craving: _____
_____

Probably because: _____
_____
_____

My Food Journal for _____ 20_____

Breakfast: _____ AM/PM home/work/school/car/other
I had _____
_____
Proud that I DID NOT have: _____

Snack #1: _____ AM/PM home/work/school/car/other
I had _____
_____
Proud that I DID NOT have: _____

Lunch: _____ AM/PM home/work/school/car/other
I had _____
_____
Proud that I DID NOT have: _____

Snack #2: _____ AM/PM home/work/school/car/other
I had _____
_____
Proud that I DID NOT have: _____

Dinner: _____ AM/PM home/work/school/car/other
I had _____
_____
Proud that I DID NOT have: _____

Drank ___1 ___2 ___3 ___4 ___5 ___6 ___7 ___8 glasses of water!

And feel GOOD about: _____
_____

Weight Loss Worksheet for _____ 20_____

Today is Day _____ of 30 and I weigh _____ at _____ am/pm

I have completed a total of _____ minutes of exercise
Including _____
_____

I have eliminated the following garbage food from my diet:
_____
_____

I have replaced the junk with these healthier food choices:
_____
_____

I am particularly proud of Today's accomplishments:
_____
_____

And the ways that I handled stress: _____
_____
_____

But I am REALLY craving: _____
_____

Probably because: _____
_____
_____

My Food Journal for _____ 20_____

Breakfast: _____ AM/PM home/work/school/car/other
I had _____
_____
Proud that I DID NOT have: _____

Snack #1: _____ AM/PM home/work/school/car/other
I had _____
_____
Proud that I DID NOT have: _____

Lunch: _____ AM/PM home/work/school/car/other
I had _____
_____
Proud that I DID NOT have: _____

Snack #2: _____ AM/PM home/work/school/car/other
I had _____
_____
Proud that I DID NOT have: _____

Dinner: _____ AM/PM home/work/school/car/other
I had _____
_____
Proud that I DID NOT have: _____

Drank ___1 ___2 ___3 ___4 ___5 ___6 ___7 ___8 glasses of water!

And feel GOOD about: _____
_____

Weight Loss Worksheet for _____ 20_____

Today is Day _____ of 30 and I weigh _____ at _____ am/pm

I have completed a total of _____ minutes of exercise
Including _____
_____

I have eliminated the following garbage food from my diet:
_____
_____

I have replaced the junk with these healthier food choices:
_____
_____

I am particularly proud of Today's accomplishments:
_____
_____

And the ways that I handled stress: _____
_____
_____

But I am REALLY craving: _____
_____

Probably because: _____
_____
_____

My Food Journal for _____ 20_____

Breakfast: _____ AM/PM home/work/school/car/other
I had _____
_____
Proud that I DID NOT have: _____

Snack #1: _____ AM/PM home/work/school/car/other
I had _____
_____
Proud that I DID NOT have: _____

Lunch: _____ AM/PM home/work/school/car/other
I had _____
_____
Proud that I DID NOT have: _____

Snack #2: _____ AM/PM home/work/school/car/other
I had _____
_____
Proud that I DID NOT have: _____

Dinner: _____ AM/PM home/work/school/car/other
I had _____
_____
Proud that I DID NOT have: _____

Drank ___1 ___2 ___3 ___4 ___5 ___6 ___7 ___8 glasses of water!

And feel GOOD about: _____
_____

Weight Loss Worksheet for _____ 20_____

Today is Day _____ of 30 and I weigh _____ at _____ am/pm

I have completed a total of _____ minutes of exercise
Including _____
_____

I have eliminated the following garbage food from my diet:
_____
_____

I have replaced the junk with these healthier food choices:
_____
_____

I am particularly proud of Today's accomplishments:
_____
_____

And the ways that I handled stress: _____
_____
_____

But I am REALLY craving: _____
_____

Probably because: _____
_____
_____

My Food Journal for _____ 20_____

Breakfast: _____ AM/PM home/work/school/car/other
I had _____
_____
Proud that I DID NOT have: _____

Snack #1: _____ AM/PM home/work/school/car/other
I had _____
_____
Proud that I DID NOT have: _____

Lunch: _____ AM/PM home/work/school/car/other
I had _____
_____
Proud that I DID NOT have: _____

Snack #2: _____ AM/PM home/work/school/car/other
I had _____
_____
Proud that I DID NOT have: _____

Dinner: _____ AM/PM home/work/school/car/other
I had _____
_____
Proud that I DID NOT have: _____

Drank ___1 ___2 ___3 ___4 ___5 ___6 ___7 ___8 glasses of water!

And feel GOOD about: _____
_____

Weight Loss Worksheet for _____ 20_____

Today is Day _____ of 30 and I weigh _____ at _____ am/pm

I have completed a total of _____ minutes of exercise
Including _____
_____

I have eliminated the following garbage food from my diet:
_____
_____

I have replaced the junk with these healthier food choices:
_____
_____

I am particularly proud of Today's accomplishments:
_____
_____

And the ways that I handled stress: _____
_____
_____

But I am REALLY craving: _____
_____

Probably because: _____
_____
_____

My Food Journal for _____ 20_____

Breakfast: _____ AM/PM home/work/school/car/other
I had _____
_____
Proud that I DID NOT have: _____

Snack #1: _____ AM/PM home/work/school/car/other
I had _____
_____
Proud that I DID NOT have: _____

Lunch: _____ AM/PM home/work/school/car/other
I had _____
_____
Proud that I DID NOT have: _____

Snack #2: _____ AM/PM home/work/school/car/other
I had _____
_____
Proud that I DID NOT have: _____

Dinner: _____ AM/PM home/work/school/car/other
I had _____
_____
Proud that I DID NOT have: _____

Drank ___1 ___2 ___3 ___4 ___5 ___6 ___7 ___8 glasses of water!

And feel GOOD about: _____
_____

Weight Loss Worksheet for _____ 20_____

Today is Day _____ of 30 and I weigh _____ at _____ am/pm

I have completed a total of _____ minutes of exercise
Including _____
_____

I have eliminated the following garbage food from my diet:
_____
_____

I have replaced the junk with these healthier food choices:
_____
_____

I am particularly proud of Today's accomplishments:
_____
_____

And the ways that I handled stress: _____
_____
_____

But I am REALLY craving: _____
_____

Probably because: _____
_____
_____

My Food Journal for _____ 20_____

Breakfast: _____ AM/PM home/work/school/car/other
I had _____
_____
Proud that I DID NOT have: _____

Snack #1: _____ AM/PM home/work/school/car/other
I had _____
_____
Proud that I DID NOT have: _____

Lunch: _____ AM/PM home/work/school/car/other
I had _____
_____
Proud that I DID NOT have: _____

Snack #2: _____ AM/PM home/work/school/car/other
I had _____
_____
Proud that I DID NOT have: _____

Dinner: _____ AM/PM home/work/school/car/other
I had _____
_____
Proud that I DID NOT have: _____

Drank __1 __2 __3 __4 __5 __6 __7 __8 glasses of water!

And feel GOOD about: _____
_____

Weight Loss Worksheet for _____ 20_____

Today is Day _____ of 30 and I weigh _____ at _____ am/pm

I have completed a total of _____ minutes of exercise
Including _____
_____

I have eliminated the following garbage food from my diet:
_____
_____

I have replaced the junk with these healthier food choices:
_____
_____

I am particularly proud of Today's accomplishments:
_____
_____

And the ways that I handled stress: _____
_____
_____

But I am REALLY craving: _____
_____

Probably because: _____
_____
_____

My Food Journal for _____ 20_____

Breakfast: _____ AM/PM home/work/school/car/other
I had _____
_____
Proud that I DID NOT have: _____

Snack #1: _____ AM/PM home/work/school/car/other
I had _____
_____
Proud that I DID NOT have: _____

Lunch: _____ AM/PM home/work/school/car/other
I had _____
_____
Proud that I DID NOT have: _____

Snack #2: _____ AM/PM home/work/school/car/other
I had _____
_____
Proud that I DID NOT have: _____

Dinner: _____ AM/PM home/work/school/car/other
I had _____
_____
Proud that I DID NOT have: _____

Drank __1 __2 __3 __4 __5 __6 __7 __8 glasses of water!

And feel GOOD about: _____
_____

Weight Loss Worksheet for _____ 20_____

Today is Day _____ of 30 and I weigh _____ at _____ am/pm

I have completed a total of _____ minutes of exercise
Including _____
_____

I have eliminated the following garbage food from my diet:
_____
_____

I have replaced the junk with these healthier food choices:
_____
_____

I am particularly proud of Today's accomplishments:
_____
_____

And the ways that I handled stress: _____
_____
_____

But I am REALLY craving: _____
_____

Probably because: _____
_____
_____

My Food Journal for _____ 20_____

Breakfast: _____ AM/PM home/work/school/car/other
I had _____
_____
Proud that I DID NOT have: _____

Snack #1: _____ AM/PM home/work/school/car/other
I had _____
_____
Proud that I DID NOT have: _____

Lunch: _____ AM/PM home/work/school/car/other
I had _____
_____
Proud that I DID NOT have: _____

Snack #2: _____ AM/PM home/work/school/car/other
I had _____
_____
Proud that I DID NOT have: _____

Dinner: _____ AM/PM home/work/school/car/other
I had _____
_____
Proud that I DID NOT have: _____

Drank ___1 ___2 ___3 ___4 ___5 ___6 ___7 ___8 glasses of water!

And feel GOOD about: _____
_____

Weight Loss Worksheet for _____ 20_____

Today is Day _____ of 30 and I weigh _____ at _____ am/pm

I have completed a total of _____ minutes of exercise
Including _____
_____

I have eliminated the following garbage food from my diet:
_____
_____

I have replaced the junk with these healthier food choices:
_____
_____

I am particularly proud of Today's accomplishments:
_____
_____

And the ways that I handled stress: _____
_____
_____

But I am REALLY craving: _____
_____

Probably because: _____
_____
_____

My Food Journal for _____ 20_____

Breakfast: _____ AM/PM home/work/school/car/other
I had _____
_____

Proud that I DID NOT have: _____

Snack #1: _____ AM/PM home/work/school/car/other
I had _____
_____

Proud that I DID NOT have: _____

Lunch: _____ AM/PM home/work/school/car/other
I had _____
_____

Proud that I DID NOT have: _____

Snack #2: _____ AM/PM home/work/school/car/other
I had _____
_____

Proud that I DID NOT have: _____

Dinner: _____ AM/PM home/work/school/car/other
I had _____
_____

Proud that I DID NOT have: _____

Drank ___1 ___2 ___3 ___4 ___5 ___6 ___7 ___8 glasses of water!

And feel GOOD about: _____
_____

Weight Loss Worksheet for _____ 20_____

Today is Day _____ of 30 and I weigh _____ at _____ am/pm

I have completed a total of _____ minutes of exercise
Including _____
_____

I have eliminated the following garbage food from my diet:
_____
_____

I have replaced the junk with these healthier food choices:
_____
_____

I am particularly proud of Today's accomplishments:
_____
_____

And the ways that I handled stress: _____
_____
_____

But I am REALLY craving: _____
_____

Probably because: _____
_____
_____

My Food Journal for _____ 20_____

Breakfast: _____ AM/PM home/work/school/car/other
I had _____
_____
Proud that I DID NOT have: _____

Snack #1: _____ AM/PM home/work/school/car/other
I had _____
_____
Proud that I DID NOT have: _____

Lunch: _____ AM/PM home/work/school/car/other
I had _____
_____
Proud that I DID NOT have: _____

Snack #2: _____ AM/PM home/work/school/car/other
I had _____
_____
Proud that I DID NOT have: _____

Dinner: _____ AM/PM home/work/school/car/other
I had _____
_____
Proud that I DID NOT have: _____

Drank __1 __2 __3 __4 __5 __6 __7 __8 glasses of water!

And feel GOOD about: _____
_____

Weight Loss Worksheet for _____ 20_____

Today is Day _____ of 30 and I weigh _____ at _____ am/pm

I have completed a total of _____ minutes of exercise
Including _____
_____

I have eliminated the following garbage food from my diet:
_____
_____

I have replaced the junk with these healthier food choices:
_____
_____

I am particularly proud of Today's accomplishments:
_____
_____

And the ways that I handled stress: _____
_____
_____

But I am REALLY craving: _____
_____

Probably because: _____
_____
_____

My Food Journal for _____ 20_____

Breakfast: _____ AM/PM home/work/school/car/other
I had _____
_____
Proud that I DID NOT have: _____

Snack #1: _____ AM/PM home/work/school/car/other
I had _____
_____
Proud that I DID NOT have: _____

Lunch: _____ AM/PM home/work/school/car/other
I had _____
_____
Proud that I DID NOT have: _____

Snack #2: _____ AM/PM home/work/school/car/other
I had _____
_____
Proud that I DID NOT have: _____

Dinner: _____ AM/PM home/work/school/car/other
I had _____
_____
Proud that I DID NOT have: _____

Drank ___1 ___2 ___3 ___4 ___5 ___6 ___7 ___8 glasses of water!

And feel GOOD about: _____
_____

Weight Loss Worksheet for _____ 20_____

Today is Day _____ of 30 and I weigh _____ at _____ am/pm

I have completed a total of _____ minutes of exercise
Including _____
_____

I have eliminated the following garbage food from my diet:
_____
_____

I have replaced the junk with these healthier food choices:
_____
_____

I am particularly proud of Today's accomplishments:
_____
_____

And the ways that I handled stress: _____
_____
_____

But I am REALLY craving: _____
_____

Probably because: _____
_____
_____

My Food Journal for _____ 20_____

Breakfast: _____ AM/PM home/work/school/car/other
I had _____

_____
Proud that I DID NOT have: _____

Snack #1: _____ AM/PM home/work/school/car/other
I had _____

_____
Proud that I DID NOT have: _____

Lunch: _____ AM/PM home/work/school/car/other
I had _____

_____
Proud that I DID NOT have: _____

Snack #2: _____ AM/PM home/work/school/car/other
I had _____

_____
Proud that I DID NOT have: _____

Dinner: _____ AM/PM home/work/school/car/other
I had _____

_____
Proud that I DID NOT have: _____

Drank ___1 ___2 ___3 ___4 ___5 ___6 ___7 ___8 glasses of water!

And feel GOOD about: _____

_____

Weight Loss Worksheet for _____ 20_____

Today is Day _____ of 30 and I weigh _____ at _____ am/pm

I have completed a total of _____ minutes of exercise
Including _____
_____

I have eliminated the following garbage food from my diet:
_____
_____

I have replaced the junk with these healthier food choices:
_____
_____

I am particularly proud of Today's accomplishments:
_____
_____

And the ways that I handled stress: _____
_____
_____

But I am REALLY craving: _____
_____

Probably because: _____
_____
_____

My Food Journal for _____ 20_____

Breakfast: _____ AM/PM home/work/school/car/other
I had _____
_____
Proud that I DID NOT have: _____

Snack #1: _____ AM/PM home/work/school/car/other
I had _____
_____
Proud that I DID NOT have: _____

Lunch: _____ AM/PM home/work/school/car/other
I had _____
_____
Proud that I DID NOT have: _____

Snack #2: _____ AM/PM home/work/school/car/other
I had _____
_____
Proud that I DID NOT have: _____

Dinner: _____ AM/PM home/work/school/car/other
I had _____
_____
Proud that I DID NOT have: _____

Drank ___1 ___2 ___3 ___4 ___5 ___6 ___7 ___8 glasses of water!

And feel GOOD about: _____
_____

Weight Loss Worksheet for _____ 20_____

Today is Day _____ of 30 and I weigh _____ at _____ am/pm

I have completed a total of _____ minutes of exercise
Including _____
_____

I have eliminated the following garbage food from my diet:
_____
_____

I have replaced the junk with these healthier food choices:
_____
_____

I am particularly proud of Today's accomplishments:
_____
_____

And the ways that I handled stress: _____
_____
_____

But I am REALLY craving: _____
_____

Probably because: _____
_____
_____

My Food Journal for _____ 20_____

Breakfast: _____ AM/PM home/work/school/car/other
I had _____
_____
Proud that I DID NOT have: _____

Snack #1: _____ AM/PM home/work/school/car/other
I had _____
_____
Proud that I DID NOT have: _____

Lunch: _____ AM/PM home/work/school/car/other
I had _____
_____
Proud that I DID NOT have: _____

Snack #2: _____ AM/PM home/work/school/car/other
I had _____
_____
Proud that I DID NOT have: _____

Dinner: _____ AM/PM home/work/school/car/other
I had _____
_____
Proud that I DID NOT have: _____

Drank __1 __2 __3 __4 __5 __6 __7 __8 glasses of water!

And feel GOOD about: _____
_____

Weight Loss Worksheet for _____ 20_____

Today is Day _____ of 30 and I weigh _____ at _____ am/pm

I have completed a total of _____ minutes of exercise
Including _____
_____

I have eliminated the following garbage food from my diet:
_____
_____

I have replaced the junk with these healthier food choices:
_____
_____

I am particularly proud of Today's accomplishments:
_____
_____

And the ways that I handled stress: _____
_____
_____

But I am REALLY craving: _____
_____

Probably because: _____
_____
_____

My Food Journal for _____ 20_____

Breakfast: _____ AM/PM home/work/school/car/other
I had _____
_____
Proud that I DID NOT have: _____

Snack #1: _____ AM/PM home/work/school/car/other
I had _____
_____
Proud that I DID NOT have: _____

Lunch: _____ AM/PM home/work/school/car/other
I had _____
_____
Proud that I DID NOT have: _____

Snack #2: _____ AM/PM home/work/school/car/other
I had _____
_____
Proud that I DID NOT have: _____

Dinner: _____ AM/PM home/work/school/car/other
I had _____
_____
Proud that I DID NOT have: _____

Drank ___1 ___2 ___3 ___4 ___5 ___6 ___7 ___8 glasses of water!

And feel GOOD about: _____
_____

Weight Loss Worksheet for _____ 20_____

Today is Day _____ of 30 and I weigh _____ at _____ am/pm

I have completed a total of _____ minutes of exercise
Including _____
_____

I have eliminated the following garbage food from my diet:
_____
_____

I have replaced the junk with these healthier food choices:
_____
_____

I am particularly proud of Today's accomplishments:
_____
_____

And the ways that I handled stress: _____
_____
_____

But I am REALLY craving: _____
_____

Probably because: _____
_____
_____

My Food Journal for _____ 20_____

Breakfast: _____ AM/PM home/work/school/car/other
I had _____
_____
Proud that I DID NOT have: _____

Snack #1: _____ AM/PM home/work/school/car/other
I had _____
_____
Proud that I DID NOT have: _____

Lunch: _____ AM/PM home/work/school/car/other
I had _____
_____
Proud that I DID NOT have: _____

Snack #2: _____ AM/PM home/work/school/car/other
I had _____
_____
Proud that I DID NOT have: _____

Dinner: _____ AM/PM home/work/school/car/other
I had _____
_____
Proud that I DID NOT have: _____

Drank __1 __2 __3 __4 __5 __6 __7 __8 glasses of water!

And feel GOOD about: _____
_____

Weight Loss Worksheet for _____ 20_____

Today is Day _____ of 30 and I weigh _____ at _____ am/pm

I have completed a total of _____ minutes of exercise
Including _____
_____

I have eliminated the following garbage food from my diet:
_____
_____

I have replaced the junk with these healthier food choices:
_____
_____

I am particularly proud of Today's accomplishments:
_____
_____

And the ways that I handled stress: _____
_____
_____

But I am REALLY craving: _____
_____

Probably because: _____
_____
_____

My Food Journal for _____ 20_____

Breakfast: _____ AM/PM home/work/school/car/other
I had _____
_____
Proud that I DID NOT have: _____

Snack #1: _____ AM/PM home/work/school/car/other
I had _____
_____
Proud that I DID NOT have: _____

Lunch: _____ AM/PM home/work/school/car/other
I had _____
_____
Proud that I DID NOT have: _____

Snack #2: _____ AM/PM home/work/school/car/other
I had _____
_____
Proud that I DID NOT have: _____

Dinner: _____ AM/PM home/work/school/car/other
I had _____
_____
Proud that I DID NOT have: _____

Drank ___1 ___2 ___3 ___4 ___5 ___6 ___7 ___8 glasses of water!

And feel GOOD about: _____
_____

Weight Loss Worksheet for _____ 20_____

Today is Day _____ of 30 and I weigh _____ at _____ am/pm

I have completed a total of _____ minutes of exercise
Including _____
_____

I have eliminated the following garbage food from my diet:
_____
_____

I have replaced the junk with these healthier food choices:
_____
_____

I am particularly proud of Today's accomplishments:
_____
_____

And the ways that I handled stress: _____
_____
_____

But I am REALLY craving: _____
_____

Probably because: _____
_____
_____

My Food Journal for _____ 20_____

Breakfast: _____ AM/PM home/work/school/car/other
I had _____
_____
Proud that I DID NOT have: _____

Snack #1: _____ AM/PM home/work/school/car/other
I had _____
_____
Proud that I DID NOT have: _____

Lunch: _____ AM/PM home/work/school/car/other
I had _____
_____
Proud that I DID NOT have: _____

Snack #2: _____ AM/PM home/work/school/car/other
I had _____
_____
Proud that I DID NOT have: _____

Dinner: _____ AM/PM home/work/school/car/other
I had _____
_____
Proud that I DID NOT have: _____

Drank ___1 ___2 ___3 ___4 ___5 ___6 ___7 ___8 glasses of water!

And feel GOOD about: _____
_____

Weight Loss Worksheet for _____ 20_____

Today is Day _____ of 30 and I weigh _____ at _____ am/pm

I have completed a total of _____ minutes of exercise
Including _____
_____

I have eliminated the following garbage food from my diet:
_____
_____

I have replaced the junk with these healthier food choices:
_____
_____

I am particularly proud of Today's accomplishments:
_____
_____

And the ways that I handled stress: _____
_____
_____

But I am REALLY craving: _____
_____

Probably because: _____
_____
_____

My Food Journal for _____ 20_____

Breakfast: _____ AM/PM home/work/school/car/other
I had _____
_____
Proud that I DID NOT have: _____

Snack #1: _____ AM/PM home/work/school/car/other
I had _____
_____
Proud that I DID NOT have: _____

Lunch: _____ AM/PM home/work/school/car/other
I had _____
_____
Proud that I DID NOT have: _____

Snack #2: _____ AM/PM home/work/school/car/other
I had _____
_____
Proud that I DID NOT have: _____

Dinner: _____ AM/PM home/work/school/car/other
I had _____
_____
Proud that I DID NOT have: _____

Drank ___1 ___2 ___3 ___4 ___5 ___6 ___7 ___8 glasses of water!

And feel GOOD about: _____
_____

Weight Loss Worksheet for _____ 20_____

Today is Day _____ of 30 and I weigh _____ at _____ am/pm

I have completed a total of _____ minutes of exercise
Including _____
_____

I have eliminated the following garbage food from my diet:
_____
_____

I have replaced the junk with these healthier food choices:
_____
_____

I am particularly proud of Today's accomplishments:
_____
_____

And the ways that I handled stress: _____
_____
_____

But I am REALLY craving: _____
_____

Probably because: _____
_____
_____

My Food Journal for _____ 20_____

Breakfast: _____ AM/PM home/work/school/car/other
I had _____
_____
Proud that I DID NOT have: _____

Snack #1: _____ AM/PM home/work/school/car/other
I had _____
_____
Proud that I DID NOT have: _____

Lunch: _____ AM/PM home/work/school/car/other
I had _____
_____
Proud that I DID NOT have: _____

Snack #2: _____ AM/PM home/work/school/car/other
I had _____
_____
Proud that I DID NOT have: _____

Dinner: _____ AM/PM home/work/school/car/other
I had _____
_____
Proud that I DID NOT have: _____

Drank __1 __2 __3 __4 __5 __6 __7 __8 glasses of water!

And feel GOOD about: _____
_____

Weight Loss Worksheet for _____ 20_____

Today is Day _____ of 30 and I weigh _____ at _____ am/pm

I have completed a total of _____ minutes of exercise
Including _____
_____

I have eliminated the following garbage food from my diet:
_____
_____

I have replaced the junk with these healthier food choices:
_____
_____

I am particularly proud of Today's accomplishments:
_____
_____

And the ways that I handled stress: _____
_____
_____

But I am REALLY craving: _____
_____

Probably because: _____
_____
_____

My Food Journal for _____ 20_____

Breakfast: _____ AM/PM home/work/school/car/other
I had _____
_____
Proud that I DID NOT have: _____

Snack #1: _____ AM/PM home/work/school/car/other
I had _____
_____
Proud that I DID NOT have: _____

Lunch: _____ AM/PM home/work/school/car/other
I had _____
_____
Proud that I DID NOT have: _____

Snack #2: _____ AM/PM home/work/school/car/other
I had _____
_____
Proud that I DID NOT have: _____

Dinner: _____ AM/PM home/work/school/car/other
I had _____
_____
Proud that I DID NOT have: _____

Drank ___1 ___2 ___3 ___4 ___5 ___6 ___7 ___8 glasses of water!

And feel GOOD about: _____
_____

Weight Loss Worksheet for _____ 20_____

Today is Day _____ of 30 and I weigh _____ at _____ am/pm

I have completed a total of _____ minutes of exercise
Including _____
_____

I have eliminated the following garbage food from my diet:
_____
_____

I have replaced the junk with these healthier food choices:
_____
_____

I am particularly proud of Today's accomplishments:
_____
_____

And the ways that I handled stress: _____
_____
_____

But I am REALLY craving: _____
_____

Probably because: _____
_____
_____

My Food Journal for _____ 20_____

Breakfast: _____ AM/PM home/work/school/car/other
I had _____
_____

Proud that I DID NOT have: _____

Snack #1: _____ AM/PM home/work/school/car/other
I had _____
_____

Proud that I DID NOT have: _____

Lunch: _____ AM/PM home/work/school/car/other
I had _____
_____

Proud that I DID NOT have: _____

Snack #2: _____ AM/PM home/work/school/car/other
I had _____
_____

Proud that I DID NOT have: _____

Dinner: _____ AM/PM home/work/school/car/other
I had _____
_____

Proud that I DID NOT have: _____

Drank ___1 ___2 ___3 ___4 ___5 ___6 ___7 ___8 glasses of water!

And feel GOOD about: _____
_____

Weight Loss Worksheet for _____ 20_____

Today is Day _____ of 30 and I weigh _____ at _____ am/pm

I have completed a total of _____ minutes of exercise
Including _____
_____

I have eliminated the following garbage food from my diet:
_____
_____

I have replaced the junk with these healthier food choices:
_____
_____

I am particularly proud of Today's accomplishments:
_____
_____

And the ways that I handled stress: _____
_____
_____

But I am REALLY craving: _____
_____

Probably because: _____
_____
_____

My Food Journal for _____ 20_____

Breakfast: _____ AM/PM home/work/school/car/other
I had _____

_____
Proud that I DID NOT have: _____

Snack #1: _____ AM/PM home/work/school/car/other
I had _____

_____
Proud that I DID NOT have: _____

Lunch: _____ AM/PM home/work/school/car/other
I had _____

_____
Proud that I DID NOT have: _____

Snack #2: _____ AM/PM home/work/school/car/other
I had _____

_____
Proud that I DID NOT have: _____

Dinner: _____ AM/PM home/work/school/car/other
I had _____

_____
Proud that I DID NOT have: _____

Drank __1 __2 __3 __4 __5 __6 __7 __8 glasses of water!

And feel GOOD about: _____

_____

Weight Loss Worksheet for _____ 20_____

Today is Day _____ of 30 and I weigh _____ at _____ am/pm

I have completed a total of _____ minutes of exercise
Including _____
_____

I have eliminated the following garbage food from my diet:
_____
_____

I have replaced the junk with these healthier food choices:
_____
_____

I am particularly proud of Today's accomplishments:
_____
_____

And the ways that I handled stress: _____
_____
_____

But I am REALLY craving: _____
_____

Probably because: _____
_____
_____

My Food Journal for _____ 20_____

Breakfast: _____ AM/PM home/work/school/car/other
I had _____
_____
Proud that I DID NOT have: _____

Snack #1: _____ AM/PM home/work/school/car/other
I had _____
_____
Proud that I DID NOT have: _____

Lunch: _____ AM/PM home/work/school/car/other
I had _____
_____
Proud that I DID NOT have: _____

Snack #2: _____ AM/PM home/work/school/car/other
I had _____
_____
Proud that I DID NOT have: _____

Dinner: _____ AM/PM home/work/school/car/other
I had _____
_____
Proud that I DID NOT have: _____

Drank ___1 ___2 ___3 ___4 ___5 ___6 ___7 ___8 glasses of water!

And feel GOOD about: _____
_____

Weight Loss Worksheet for _____ 20_____

Today is Day _____ of 30 and I weigh _____ at _____ am/pm

I have completed a total of _____ minutes of exercise
Including _____
_____

I have eliminated the following garbage food from my diet:
_____
_____

I have replaced the junk with these healthier food choices:
_____
_____

I am particularly proud of Today's accomplishments:
_____
_____

And the ways that I handled stress: _____
_____
_____

But I am REALLY craving: _____
_____

Probably because: _____
_____
_____

My Food Journal for _____ 20_____

Breakfast: _____ AM/PM home/work/school/car/other
I had _____
_____
Proud that I DID NOT have: _____

Snack #1: _____ AM/PM home/work/school/car/other
I had _____
_____
Proud that I DID NOT have: _____

Lunch: _____ AM/PM home/work/school/car/other
I had _____
_____
Proud that I DID NOT have: _____

Snack #2: _____ AM/PM home/work/school/car/other
I had _____
_____
Proud that I DID NOT have: _____

Dinner: _____ AM/PM home/work/school/car/other
I had _____
_____
Proud that I DID NOT have: _____

Drank __1 __2 __3 __4 __5 __6 __7 __8 glasses of water!

And feel GOOD about: _____
_____

Weight Loss Worksheet for _____ 20_____

Today is Day _____ of 30 and I weigh _____ at _____ am/pm

I have completed a total of _____ minutes of exercise
Including _____
_____

I have eliminated the following garbage food from my diet:
_____
_____

I have replaced the junk with these healthier food choices:
_____
_____

I am particularly proud of Today's accomplishments:
_____
_____

And the ways that I handled stress: _____
_____
_____

But I am REALLY craving: _____
_____

Probably because: _____
_____
_____

My Food Journal for _____ 20_____

Breakfast: _____ AM/PM home/work/school/car/other
I had _____
_____
Proud that I DID NOT have: _____

Snack #1: _____ AM/PM home/work/school/car/other
I had _____
_____
Proud that I DID NOT have: _____

Lunch: _____ AM/PM home/work/school/car/other
I had _____
_____
Proud that I DID NOT have: _____

Snack #2: _____ AM/PM home/work/school/car/other
I had _____
_____
Proud that I DID NOT have: _____

Dinner: _____ AM/PM home/work/school/car/other
I had _____
_____
Proud that I DID NOT have: _____

Drank __1 __2 __3 __4 __5 __6 __7 __8 glasses of water!

And feel GOOD about: _____
_____

Weight Loss Worksheet for _____ 20_____

Today is Day _____ of 30 and I weigh _____ at _____ am/pm

I have completed a total of _____ minutes of exercise
Including _____
_____

I have eliminated the following garbage food from my diet:
_____
_____

I have replaced the junk with these healthier food choices:
_____
_____

I am particularly proud of Today's accomplishments:
_____
_____

And the ways that I handled stress: _____
_____
_____

But I am REALLY craving: _____
_____

Probably because: _____
_____
_____

My Food Journal for _____ 20_____

Breakfast: _____ AM/PM home/work/school/car/other
I had _____
_____
Proud that I DID NOT have: _____

Snack #1: _____ AM/PM home/work/school/car/other
I had _____
_____
Proud that I DID NOT have: _____

Lunch: _____ AM/PM home/work/school/car/other
I had _____
_____
Proud that I DID NOT have: _____

Snack #2: _____ AM/PM home/work/school/car/other
I had _____
_____
Proud that I DID NOT have: _____

Dinner: _____ AM/PM home/work/school/car/other
I had _____
_____
Proud that I DID NOT have: _____

Drank ___1 ___2 ___3 ___4 ___5 ___6 ___7 ___8 glasses of water!

And feel GOOD about: _____
_____

Weight Loss Worksheet for _____ 20_____

Today is Day _____ of 30 and I weigh _____ at _____ am/pm

I have completed a total of _____ minutes of exercise
Including ---

I have eliminated the following garbage food from my diet:

I have replaced the junk with these healthier food choices:

I am particularly proud of Today's accomplishments:

And the ways that I handled stress: _____

But I am REALLY craving: _____

Probably because: _____

My Food Journal for _____ 20_____

Breakfast: _____ AM/PM home/work/school/car/other
I had _____
_____
Proud that I DID NOT have: _____

Snack #1: _____ AM/PM home/work/school/car/other
I had _____
_____
Proud that I DID NOT have: _____

Lunch: _____ AM/PM home/work/school/car/other
I had _____
_____
Proud that I DID NOT have: _____

Snack #2: _____ AM/PM home/work/school/car/other
I had _____
_____
Proud that I DID NOT have: _____

Dinner: _____ AM/PM home/work/school/car/other
I had _____
_____
Proud that I DID NOT have: _____

Drank ___1 ___2 ___3 ___4 ___5 ___6 ___7 ___8 glasses of water!

And feel GOOD about: _____
_____

Weight Loss Worksheet for _____ 20_____

Today is Day _____ of 30 and I weigh _____ at _____ am/pm

I have completed a total of _____ minutes of exercise
Including _____
_____

I have eliminated the following garbage food from my diet:
_____
_____

I have replaced the junk with these healthier food choices:
_____
_____

I am particularly proud of Today's accomplishments:
_____
_____

And the ways that I handled stress: _____
_____
_____

But I am REALLY craving: _____
_____

Probably because: _____
_____
_____

My Food Journal for _____ 20_____

Breakfast: _____ AM/PM home/work/school/car/other
I had _____
_____
Proud that I DID NOT have: _____

Snack #1: _____ AM/PM home/work/school/car/other
I had _____
_____
Proud that I DID NOT have: _____

Lunch: _____ AM/PM home/work/school/car/other
I had _____
_____
Proud that I DID NOT have: _____

Snack #2: _____ AM/PM home/work/school/car/other
I had _____
_____
Proud that I DID NOT have: _____

Dinner: _____ AM/PM home/work/school/car/other
I had _____
_____
Proud that I DID NOT have: _____

Drank __1 __2 __3 __4 __5 __6 __7 __8 glasses of water!

And feel GOOD about: _____
_____